The Vibrant Ketogenic Cookbook for Beginners

Healthy and Tasty Recipes to Start Your Keto Diet and Stay Fit

Lauren Loose

© Copyright 2021 - All rights reserved.

The content contained within this book may not be reproduced, duplicated or transmitted without direct written permission from the author or the publisher.

Under no circumstances will any blame or legal responsibility be held against the publisher, or author, for any damages, reparation, or monetary loss due to the information contained within this book. Either directly or indirectly.

Legal Notice:

This book is copyright protected. This book is only for personal use. You cannot amend, distribute, sell, use, quote or paraphrase any part, or the content within this book, without the consent of the author or publisher.

Disclaimer Notice:

Please note the information contained within this document is for educational and entertainment purposes only. All effort has been executed to present accurate, up to date, and reliable, complete information. No warranties of any kind are declared or implied. Readers acknowledge that the author is not engaging in the rendering of legal, financial, medical or professional advice. The content within this book has been derived from various sources. Please consult a licensed professional before attempting any techniques outlined in this book.

By reading this document, the reader agrees that under no circumstances is the author responsible for any losses, direct or indirect, which are incurred as a result of the use of information contained within this document, including, but not limited to, — errors, omissions, or inaccuracies.

Contents

Mahi-Mahi Taco Wraps 8
Shrimp Scampi 10
Shrimp Tacos 12
Fish Curry 14
Salmon with Creamy Lemon Sauce 16
Salmon with   Lemon-Caper Sauce 19
Spicy Barbecue Shrimp 21
Lemon Dill Halibut 23
Coconut Cilantro Curry Shrimp 25
Shrimp in Marinara Sauce 27
Garlic Shrimp 29
Poached Salmon 31
Lemon Pepper Tilapia 33
Clam Chowder 35
Soy-Ginger Steamed Pompano 36
Ketogenic Salmon Tandoori with Cucumber Sauce 38
Creamy Mackerel 40
Lime Mackerel 41
Turmeric Tilapia 42
Walnut Salmon Mix 43
Seared Scallops Topped with Wasabi Mayo 44
Lobster-Stuffed Avocado 46
Mexican Shrimp Gazpacho 48
Manhattan Clam Chowder 51
Fried Soft-Shell Crab 54
Convenient Tilapia Casserole 56

Quick Dinner Tilapia	58
Hit Salmon Dinner	59
Luscious Salmon	61
Insanely Simple Salmon	62
Entertaining Salmon	64
Flavors Infused Salmon	66
Tuna Fish Salad	67
Mozzarella Tuna Melt	69
Crabmeat Egg Scramble with White Sauce	70
Tuna Pickle Boats	72
Salmon Salad with Lettuce & Avocado	73
Mackerel Lettuce Cups	74
Watercress & Shrimp Salad with Lemon Dressing	76
Salad of Prawns and Mixed Lettuce Greens	78
Ketogenic Baked Salmon with Lemon and Butter	80
Ketogenicgenic Spicy Oyster	82
Garlic Lime Mahi-Mahi	84
Fish and Leek Sauté	86
Smoked Salmon Salad	88
Ketogenic Baked Salmon with Pesto	90
Roasted Salmon with Parmesan Dill Crust	92
Ketogenic Fried Salmon with Broccoli and Cheese	94
Breakfast Potatoes	96
Potato Breakfast Hash	98
Tasty Potato Hash	100
Baked Potatoes	102
Whole Baked Potatoes	103

Crispy Potatoes 105
Herb Roasted New Potatoes... 107
Mashed Potatoes 109

Mahi-Mahi Taco Wraps

Preparation Time: 5 minutes

Cooking Time: 2 hours

Servings: 6

Ingredients:

- 1-pound Mahi-Mahi, wild-caught
- ½ cup cherry tomatoes
- 1 small green bell pepper, cored and sliced
- 1/4 of a medium red onion, thinly sliced
- ½ teaspoon garlic powder
- 1 teaspoon sea salt
- ½ teaspoon ground black pepper
- 1 teaspoon chipotle pepper
- ½ teaspoon dried oregano
- 1 teaspoon cumin
- 2 tablespoons avocado oil
- 1/4 cup chicken stock
- 1 medium avocado, diced
- 1 cup sour cream
- 6 large lettuce leaves

Directions:

1. Grease a 6-quarts slow cooker with oil, place fish in it and then pour in chicken stock. Stir together garlic powder, salt, black pepper,

chipotle pepper, oregano and cumin and then season fish with half of this mixture.

2. Layer fish with tomatoes, pepper and onion, season with remaining spice mixture and shut with lid. Plug in the slow cooker and cook fish for 2 hours at high heat setting or until cooked through. When done, evenly spoon fish among lettuce, top with avocado and sour cream and serve.

Nutrition:

193.6g Calories

12g Total Fat

17g Protein

3g Fiber

Shrimp Scampi

Preparation Time: 5 minutes

Cooking Time: 2 hours and 30 minutes

Servings: 4

Ingredients:

- 1 pound wild-caught shrimps, peeled & deveined
- 1 tablespoon minced garlic
- 1 teaspoon salt
- ½ teaspoon ground black pepper
- 1/2 teaspoon red pepper flakes
- 2 tablespoons chopped parsley
- 2 tablespoons avocado oil
- 2 tablespoons unsalted butter
- 1/2 cup white wine
- 1 tablespoon lemon juice
- 1/4 cup chicken broth
- ½ cup grated parmesan cheese

Directions:

1. Place all the ingredients except for shrimps and cheese in a 6-quart slow cooker and whisk until combined. Add shrimps and stir until evenly coated and shut with lid.

2. Plug in the slow cooker and cook for 1 hour and 30 minutes to 2 hours and 30 minutes at low heat setting or until cooked through. Then top with parmesan cheese and serve.

Nutrition:

234 Calories

14.7g Total Fat

23.3g Protein

Shrimp Tacos

Preparation Time: 5 minutes

Cooking Time: 3 hours

Servings: 6

Ingredients:

- 1 pound medium wild-caught shrimp, peeled and tails off
- 12-ounce fire-roasted tomatoes, diced
- 1 small green bell pepper, chopped
- ½ cup chopped white onion
- 1 teaspoon minced garlic
- ½ teaspoon sea salt
- ½ teaspoon ground black pepper
- ½ teaspoon red chili powder
- ½ teaspoon cumin
- ¼ teaspoon cayenne pepper
- 2 tablespoons avocado oil
- 1/2 cup salsa
- 4 tablespoons chopped cilantro
- 1 ½ cup sour cream
- 2 media avocados, diced

Directions:

1. Rinse shrimps, layer into a 6-quarts slow cooker and drizzle with oil. Add tomatoes, stir

until mixed, then add peppers and remaining ingredients except for sour cream and avocado and stir until combined.
2. Plug in the slow cooker, shut with lid and cook for 2 to 3 hours at low heat setting or 1 hour and 30 minutes to 2 hours at high heat setting or until shrimps turn pink. When done, serve shrimps with avocado and sour cream.

Nutrition:

369 Calories

27.5g Total Fat

21.2g Protein

Fish Curry

Preparation Time: 5 minutes

Cooking Time: 4 hours and 30 minutes

Servings: 6

Ingredients:

- 12 pounds wild-caught white fish fillet, cubed
- 18-ounce spinach leaves
- 4 tablespoons red curry paste, organic
- 14-ounce coconut cream, unsweetened and full-fat
- 14-ounce water

Directions:

1. Plug in a 6-quart slow cooker and let preheat at high heat setting. In the meantime, whisk together coconut cream and water until smooth.
2. Place fish into the slow cooker, spread with curry paste and then pour in coconut cream mixture. Shut with lid and cook for 2 hours at high heat setting or 4 hours at low heat setting until tender.
3. Then add spinach and continue cooking for 20 to 30 minutes or until spinach leaves wilt. Serve straightaway.

Nutrition:

323 Calories

51.5g Total Fat

41.3g Protein

Salmon with Creamy Lemon Sauce

Preparation Time: 5 minutes

Cooking Time: 2 hours and 15 minutes

Servings: 6

Ingredients:

For the Salmon:

- 2 pounds wild-caught salmon fillet, skin-on
- 1 teaspoon garlic powder
- 1 ½ teaspoon salt
- 1 teaspoon ground black pepper
- 1/2 teaspoon red chili powder
- 1 teaspoon Italian Seasoning
- 1 lemon, sliced
- 1 lemon, juiced
- 2 tablespoons avocado oil
- 1 cup chicken broth

For the Creamy Lemon Sauce:

- Chopped parsley, for garnish
- 1/8 teaspoon lemon zest
- 1/4 cup heavy cream
- 1/4 cup grated parmesan cheese

Directions:

Nutrition:

323 Calories

51.5g Total Fat

41.3g Protein

Salmon with Creamy Lemon Sauce

Preparation Time: 5 minutes

Cooking Time: 2 hours and 15 minutes

Servings: 6

Ingredients:

For the Salmon:

- 2 pounds wild-caught salmon fillet, skin-on
- 1 teaspoon garlic powder
- 1 ½ teaspoon salt
- 1 teaspoon ground black pepper
- 1/2 teaspoon red chili powder
- 1 teaspoon Italian Seasoning
- 1 lemon, sliced
- 1 lemon, juiced
- 2 tablespoons avocado oil
- 1 cup chicken broth

For the Creamy Lemon Sauce:

- Chopped parsley, for garnish
- 1/8 teaspoon lemon zest
- 1/4 cup heavy cream
- 1/4 cup grated parmesan cheese

Directions:

1. Line a 6-quart slow cooker with parchment sheet, spread its bottom with lemon slices, then top with salmon and drizzle with oil. Stir together garlic powder, salt, black pepper, red chili powder, Italian seasoning, and oil until combined and rub this mixture all over salmon.
2. Pour lemon juice and broth around the fish and shut with lid. Plug in the slow cooker and cook for 2 hours at low heat setting. In the meantime, set the oven at 400 degrees F and let preheat.
3. When fish is done, lift out an inner pot of slow cooker, place into the oven and cook for 5 to 8 minutes or until top is nicely browned. Lift out fish using parchment sheet and keep it warm.
4. Transfer juices from slow cooker to a medium skillet pan, place it over medium-high heat, then bring to boil and cook for 1 minute. Turn heat to a low level, whisk cream into the sauce along with lemon zest and parmesan cheese and cook for 2 to 3 minutes or until thickened. Cut salmon in pieces, then top each piece with lemon sauce and serve.

Nutrition:

340 Calories

20g Total Fat

32g Protein

Salmon with Lemon-Caper Sauce

Preparation Time: 5 minutes

Cooking Time: 1 hour and 30 minutes

Servings: 4

Ingredients:

- 1 pound wild-caught salmon fillet
- 2 teaspoon capers, rinsed and mashed
- 1 teaspoon minced garlic
- 1 teaspoon salt
- ½ teaspoon ground black pepper
- 1/2 teaspoon dried oregano
- 1 teaspoon lemon zest
- 2 tablespoons lemon juice
- 4 tablespoons unsalted butter

Directions:

1. Cut salmon into 4 pieces, then season with salt and black pepper and sprinkle lemon zest on top. Line a 6-quart slow cooker with parchment paper, place seasoned salmon pieces on it and shut with lid.
2. Plug in the slow cooker and cook for 1 hour and 30 minutes or until salmon is cooked through. When 10 minutes of cooking time is left,

prepare lemon-caper sauce and for this, place a small saucepan over low heat, add butter and let it melt.

3. Then add capers, garlic, lemon juice, stir until mixed and simmer for 1 minute. Remove saucepan from heat and stir in oregano. When salmon is cooked, spoon lemon-caper sauce on it and serve.

Nutrition:

368.5 Calories

26.6g Total Fat

19.5g Protein

Spicy Barbecue Shrimp

Preparation Time: 5 minutes

Cooking Time: 1 hour and 30 minutes

Servings: 6

Ingredients:

- 1 1/2 pounds large wild-caught shrimp, unpeeled
- 1 green onion, chopped
- 1 teaspoon minced garlic
- 1 ½ teaspoon salt
- ¾ teaspoon ground black pepper
- 1 teaspoon Cajun seasoning
- 1 tablespoon hot pepper sauce
- ¼ cup Worcestershire Sauce
- 1 lemon, juiced
- 2 tablespoons avocado oil
- 1/2 cup unsalted butter, chopped

Directions:

1. Place all the ingredients except for shrimps in a 6-quart slow cooker and whisk until mixed. Plug in the slow cooker, then shut with lid and cook for 30 minutes at high heat setting. Then take out ½ cup of this sauce and reserve. Add shrimps to slow cooker.

Nutrition:

321 Calories

21.4g Total Fat

27.3g Protein

Lemon Dill Halibut

Preparation Time: 5 minutes

Cooking Time: 2 hours

Servings: 2

Ingredients:

- 12-ounce wild-caught halibut fillet
- 1 teaspoon salt
- ½ teaspoon ground black pepper
- 1 1/2 teaspoon dried dill
- 1 tablespoon fresh lemon juice
- 3 tablespoons avocado oil

Directions:

1. Cut an 18-inch piece of aluminum foil, place halibut fillet in the middle and then season with salt and black pepper. Whisk together remaining ingredients, drizzle this mixture over halibut, then crimp the edges of foil and place it into a 6-quart slow cooker.
2. Plug in the slow cooker, shut with lid and cook for 1 hour and 30 minutes or 2 hours at high heat setting or until cooked through. When done, carefully open the crimped edges and check the fish, it should be tender and flaky. Serve straightaway.

Nutrition:

321.5 Calories

21.4g Total Fat

32.1g Protein

Coconut Cilantro Curry Shrimp

Preparation Time: 5 minutes

Cooking Time: 2 hours and 30 minutes

Servings: 4

Ingredients:

- 1 pound wild-caught shrimp, peeled and deveined
- 2 ½ teaspoon lemon garlic seasoning
- 2 tablespoons red curry paste
- 4 tablespoons chopped cilantro
- 30 ounces coconut milk, unsweetened
- 16 ounces water

Directions:

1. Whisk together all the ingredients except for shrimps and 2 tablespoons cilantro and add to a 4-quart slow cooker. Plug in the slow cooker, shut with lid and cook for 2 hours at high heat setting or 4 hours at low heat setting.
2. Then add shrimps, toss until evenly coated and cook for 20 to 30 minutes at high heat settings or until shrimps are pink. Garnish shrimps with remaining cilantro and serve.

Nutrition:

160.7 Calories

8.2g Total Fat

19.3g Protein

Shrimp in Marinara Sauce

Preparation Time: 5 minutes

Cooking Time: 5 hours and 10 minutes

Servings: 5

Ingredients:

- 1 pound cooked wild-caught shrimps, peeled and deveined
- 14.5-ounce crushed tomatoes
- ½ teaspoon minced garlic
- 1 teaspoon salt
- 1/2 teaspoon seasoned salt
- ¼ teaspoon ground black pepper
- ½ teaspoon crushed red pepper flakes
- 1/2 teaspoon dried basil
- 1/2 teaspoon dried oregano
- ½ tablespoons avocado oil
- 6-ounce chicken broth
- 2 tablespoon minced parsley
- 1/2 cup grated Parmesan cheese

Directions:

1. Place all the ingredients except for shrimps, parsley, and cheese in a 4-quart slow cooker and stir well. Then plug in the slow cooker, shut

with lid and cook for 4 to 5 hours at low heat setting.
2. Then add shrimps and parsley, stir until mixed and cook for 10 minutes at high heat setting. Garnish shrimps with cheese and serve.

Nutrition:

358.8 Calories

25.1g Total Fat

26g Protein

Garlic Shrimp

Preparation Time: 5 minutes

Cooking Time: 1 hour

Servings: 5

Ingredients:

For the Garlic Shrimp:

- 1 1/2 pounds large wild-caught shrimp, peeled and deveined
- 1/4 teaspoon ground black pepper
- 1/8 teaspoon ground cayenne pepper
- 2 ½ teaspoons minced garlic
- 1/4 cup avocado oil
- 4 tablespoons unsalted butter

For the Seasoning:

- 1 teaspoon onion powder
- 1 tablespoon garlic powder
- 1 tablespoon salt
- 2 teaspoons ground black pepper
- 1 tablespoon paprika
- 1 teaspoon cayenne pepper
- 1 teaspoon dried oregano
- 1 teaspoon dried thyme

Directions:

1. Stir together all the ingredients for seasoning, garlic, oil, and butter and add to a 4-quart slow cooker. Plug in the slow cooker, shut with lid and cook for 25 to 30 minutes at high heat setting or until cooked.
2. Then add shrimps, toss until evenly coated and continue cooking for 20 to 30 minutes at high heat setting or until shrimps are pink. When done, transfer shrimps to a serving plate, top with sauce and serve.

Nutrition:

233.6 Calories

11.7g Total Fat

30.9g Protein

Poached Salmon

Preparation Time: 5 minutes

Cooking Time: 3 hours and 35 minutes

Servings: 4

Ingredients:

- 4 steaks of wild-caught salmon
- 1 medium white onion, peeled and sliced
- 2 teaspoons minced garlic
- 1/2 teaspoon salt
- 1/8 teaspoon ground white pepper
- 1/2 teaspoon dried dill weed
- 2 tablespoons avocado oil
- 2 tablespoons unsalted butter
- 2 tablespoons lemon juice
- 1 cup water

Directions:

1. Place butter in a 4-quart slow cooker, then add salmon and drizzle with oil. Place remaining ingredients in a medium saucepan, stir until mixed and bring the mixture to boil over high heat.
2. Then pour this mixture all over salmon and shut with lid. Plug in the slow cooker and cook salmon for 3 hours and 30 minutes at low heat

setting or until salmon is tender. Serve straightaway.

Nutrition:

310 Calories

20g Total Fat

30.2g Protein

Lemon Pepper Tilapia

Preparation Time: 5 minutes

Cooking Time: 3 hours

Servings: 6

Ingredients:

- 6 wild-caught Tilapia fillets
- 4 teaspoons lemon-pepper seasoning, divided
- 6 tablespoons unsalted butter, divided
- 1/2 cup lemon juice, fresh

Directions:

1. Cut a large piece of aluminum foil for each fillet and then arrange them on a clean working space. Place each fillet in the middle of the foil, then season with lemon-pepper seasoning, drizzle with lemon juice and top with 1 tablespoon butter.
2. Gently crimp the edges of foil to form a packet and place it into a 6-quart slow cooker. Plug in the slow cooker, shut with lid and cook for 3 hours at high heat setting or until cooked through.
3. When done, carefully remove packets from the slow cooker and open the crimped edges and

check the fish, it should be tender and flaky. Serve straightaway.

Nutrition:

201.1 Calories

12.9g Total Fat

19.6g Protein

Clam Chowder

Preparation Time: 5 minutes

Cooking Time: 6 hours

Servings: 6

Ingredients:

- 20-ounce wild-caught baby clams, with juice
- ½ cup chopped scallion
- ½ cup chopped celery
- 1 teaspoon salt
- 1 teaspoon ground black pepper
- 1 teaspoon dried thyme
- 1 tablespoon avocado oil
- 2 cups coconut cream, full-fat
- 2 cups chicken broth

Directions:

1. Grease a 6-quart slow cooker with oil, then add ingredients and stir until mixed. Plug in the slow cooker, shut with lid and cook for 4 to 6 hours at low heat setting or until cooked through. Serve straightaway.

Nutrition:

357 Calories

28.9g Total Fat

15.2g Protein

Soy-Ginger Steamed Pompano

Preparation Time: 5 minutes

Cooking Time: 1 hour

Servings: 4

Ingredients:

- 1 wild-caught whole pompano, gutted and scaled
- 1 bunch scallion, diced
- 1 bunch cilantro, chopped
- 3 teaspoons minced garlic
- 1 tablespoon grated ginger
- 1 tablespoon swerve sweetener
- ¼ cup soy sauce
- ¼ cup white wine
- ¼ cup sesame oil

Directions:

1. Place scallions in a 6-quart slow cooker and top with fish. Whisk together remaining ingredients, except for cilantro, and pour the mixture all over the fish.
2. Plug in the slow cooker, shut with lid and cook for 1 hour at high heat setting or until cooked through. Garnish with cilantro and serve

Nutrition:

202.5 Calories

24.2g Total Fat

22.7g Protein

Ketogenic Salmon Tandoori with Cucumber Sauce

Preparation Time: 10 minutes

Cooking Time: 20 minutes

Servings: 4

Ingredients

- 25 ounces salmon
- Two tablespoons coconut oil
- One tablespoon tandoori seasoning

For the cucumber sauce

- 1/2 shredded cucumber
- Juice of 1/2 lime
- Two minced garlic cloves
- 1 1/4 cups sour cream

For the crispy salad

- 3 1/2 ounces lettuce
- Three scallions
- Two avocados
- One yellow bell pepper
- Juice of 1 lime

Directions:

1. Preheat the oven to 350 degrees Fahrenheit
2. Mix the tandoori seasoning with oil and coat the salmon pieces with this mixture.
3. Bake for 20 minutes

4. Place the shredded cucumber in it. Add the mayonnaise, minced garlic, and salt to the shredded cucumber.
5. Mix the lettuce, scallions, avocados, and bell pepper. Drizzle the contents with the lime juice.
6. Transfer the veggie salad to a plate and place the baked salmon over it. Top with cucumber sauce.

Nutrition:

847 Calories

73g Fat

35g Protein

Creamy Mackerel

Preparation Time: 10 minutes

Cooking Time: 20 minutes

Servings: 4

Ingredients:

- Two shallots
- Two spring onions
- Two tablespoons olive oil
- Four mackerel fillets
- 1 cup heavy cream
- One teaspoon cumin
- ½ teaspoon oregano
- Two tablespoons chives

Directions:

1. Preheat pan with the oil over medium heat, sauté spring onions and the shallots for 5 minutes.
2. Cook fish for 4 minutes.
3. Simmer the rest of the ingredients for 10 minutes more, and serve.

Nutrition:

403 Calories

33.9g Fat

22g Protein

Lime Mackerel

Preparation Time: 10 minutes

Cooking Time: 30 Minutes

Servings: 4

Ingredients:

- Four mackerel fillets
- Two tablespoons lime juice
- Two tablespoons olive oil
- ½ teaspoon sweet paprika

Directions:

1. Arrange the mackerel on a baking sheet lined with parchment paper, add the oil and the other ingredients, rub gently, and bake at 360 degrees F for 30 minutes.

Nutrition:

297 Calories

22.7g Fat

0.2g Fiber

Turmeric Tilapia

Preparation Time: 10 minutes

Cooking Time: 12 minutes

Servings: 4

Ingredients:

- Four tilapia fillets
- Two tablespoons olive oil
- One teaspoon turmeric powder
- Two spring onions
- ¼ teaspoon basil
- ¼ teaspoon garlic powder
- One tablespoon parsley

Directions:

1. Cook oil over medium heat, cook the spring onions for 2 minutes.
2. Cook fish, turmeric, and the other ingredients for 5 minutes on each side, and serve.

Nutrition:

205 Calories

8.6g Fat

0.4g Fiber

Walnut Salmon Mix

Preparation Time: 10 minutes

Cooking Time: 14 minutes

Servings: 4

Ingredients:

- Four salmon fillets
- Two tablespoons avocado oil
- One tablespoon lime juice
- Two shallots, chopped
- Two tablespoons walnuts
- Two tablespoons parsley

Directions:

1. Heat up oil over medium-high heat, sauté the shallots.
2. Add the fish and the other ingredients, cook for 6 minutes on each side, and serve.

Nutrition:

273 Calories

14.2g Fat

0.7g Fiber

Seared Scallops Topped with Wasabi Mayo

Preparation Time: 10 minutes

Cooking Time: 10 minutes

Servings: 2

Ingredients:

- 1 tsp. wasabi paste
- 1 tsp. water
- 1 tbsp. butter
- 2 tbsp. mayonnaise
- 2 slices ginger (pickled, chopped)
- 8 large sea scallops
- black pepper
- chives (chopped)
- salt

Directions:

1. Combine the wasabi paste and mayonnaise and mix well to incorporate. Use a paper towel to pat the scallops dry and season with salt and pepper.
2. In a skillet, heat the butter over medium-high heat. When the butter starts to brown, add the scallops and sear for about 1 ½ minute on each side. Place the scallops on two plates—4

scallops each—and add a dollop of wasabi mayo.
3. Finalize by topping with pickled ginger and fresh chives. Serve immediately.

Nutrition:

281 Calories

17.1g Fats

23.38g Protein

Lobster-Stuffed Avocado

Preparation Time: 15 minutes

Cooking Time: 5 minutes

Serving: 4

Ingredients:

- 1 tbsp. avocado oil mayonnaise
- 1 tbsp. lemon juice (fresh)
- 2 tbsp. butter (melted)
- 2 cups lobster meat (chopped, cooled at room temperature)
- 2 California avocados (halved, pitted)
- 1 celery stalk (chopped)
- 1 green onion (chopped)
- black pepper
- chives (fresh, chopped)
- salt

Directions:

1. In a bowl, combine the lobster meat, green onion, and celery. Add the mayonnaise, lemon juice, and butter, then toss lightly to coat evenly. Season with salt and pepper.
2. Use a spoon to scoop out some of the avocado flesh. Just leave about half an inch of flesh Spoon the lobster mixture into the avocado

halves—about half a cup for each. Garnish with chives and serve immediately.

Nutrition:

269 Calories

18.17g Fats

6.91g Carbohydrates

17.73g Protein

Mexican Shrimp Gazpacho

Preparation Time: 3 hours and 15 minutes

Cooking Time: 45 minutes

Serving: 4

Ingredients:

For the soup:

- ½ tsp. cumin
- 1 tbsp. balsamic vinegar
- ½ cup olive oil
- 5 ½ cups tomatoes (on the vine)
- 1 garlic clove
- 1 jalapeño
- 1 lime (juiced)
- 1 medium-sized cucumber
- 1 medium-sized red onion
- ½ red bell pepper
- sea salt

For the shrimp:

- ½ tsp. garlic powder
- ½ tsp. paprika
- ½ tsp. sea salt
- ½ tbsp. olive oil
- ½ lb. shrimp (peeled, deveined)
- For the toppings:

- 2 tbsp. cucumber (diced)
- 2 tbsp. red onion (minced)
- 2 tbsp. tomato (diced)
- 1 jalapeño (sliced thinly)
- 1 medium-sized avocado (sliced)

Directions:

1. Roughly chop the soup vegetables then place in a blender. Add the cumin, balsamic vinegar, and lime juice, then blend until you achieve a smooth consistency.
2. Keep the blender running on low, remove the lid, and pour the olive oil slowly until the consistency becomes creamy. Season with sea salt, transfer the soup to a different container, and chill for a minimum of 3 hours.
3. Prepare the shrimp right before serving the gazpacho. In a small bowl, combine all of the shrimp ingredients and toss lightly to coat evenly. Heat a skillet over medium-high heat, add the shrimps, and cook for about 3 to 4 minutes each side.
4. Take the soup out of the refrigerator, spoon into bowls, and top with the shrimp. Finish it off

by adding the cucumber, red onion, tomato, jalapeño, and avocado, then serve.

Nutrition:

12.2g Protein

37.2g Fat

445 Calories

Manhattan Clam Chowder

Preparation Time: 30 minutes

Cooking Time: 15 minutes

Serving: 8

Ingredients:

- ½ tsp. thyme (dried)
- 2 tbsp. tomato paste
- 6 tbsp. butter
- ¼ cup parsley (fresh, chopped)
- ½ cup bell pepper (diced)
- ½ cup carrot (chopped)
- ½ cup dry white wine
- ½ cup onion (diced)
- 1 cup clam juice
- 1 ¼ cup celery root (peeled, diced)
- 1 ¾ cup plum tomatoes (whole with juice)
- 2 ½ cup whole baby clams (canned with liquid)
- 4 cups chicken broth (unsalted)
- 1/3 lb. bacon (diced)
- 2 bay leaves
- 2 large garlic cloves (roughly chopped)
- black pepper
- salt

Directions:

1. Heat a soup pot over medium heat. Once hot, add a small amount of oil along with the diced bacon. Cook the bacon until crispy, stirring occasionally for about 5 minutes. Turn down the heat to medium-low then add bell pepper, carrot, onion, celery root, and garlic. Continue stirring to evenly coat the veggies with bacon grease.
2. Add the wine and cover the pot. Allow the veggies to sweat for 2 to 3 minutes. Open the lid, stir, then add in the bay leaves, tomato paste, and thyme. Crush the tomatoes and add them to the pot with the liquid. Also, add the clam juice and chicken broth.
3. Turn up the heat to medium-high and bring the chowder to a boil. Once it starts boiling, return the heat to medium-low and allow the chowder to simmer for about 15 minutes. Add the clams and continue simmering. Also, add the butter and stir until melted.
4. Add salt and a lot of pepper to bring out the soup's savory flavor. Finally, stir the parsley in, then serve hot.

Nutrition:

15g Protein

36.1g Fat

429 Calories

Fried Soft-Shell Crab

Preparation Time: 16 minutes

Cooking Time: 5 minutes

Serving: 2

Ingredients:

- 4 tbsp. barbecue sauce
- ½ cup lard
- ½ cup parmesan cheese (powdered)
- 2 eggs (beaten)
- 8 soft shell crabs

Directions:

1. Heat a skillet with lard over medium-high heat. Use a paper towel to pat the crabs dry. Prepare the parmesan and eggs by placing them in separate shallow dishes.
2. Dip one crab into the egg, tap off any excess, and dip into the parmesan cheese. Make sure the crab is coated well and evenly. Drop batches of crabs into the oil and cook for about 2 minutes on each side.
3. Serve the crabs hot with barbecue sauce for dipping.

Nutrition:

20.5g Protein

21.2g Fat

299 Calories

Convenient Tilapia Casserole

Preparation Time: 15 minutes

Cooking Time: 14 minutes

Serving: 4

Ingredients:

- 2 (14-oz.) cans sugar-free diced tomatoes with basil and garlic with juice
- 1/3 C. fresh parsley, chopped and divided
- ¼ tsp. dried oregano
- ½ tsp. red pepper flakes, crushed
- 4 (6-oz.) tilapia fillets
- 2 tbsp. fresh lemon juice
- 2/3 C. feta cheese, crumbled

Directions:

1. Preheat the oven to 4000 F. In a shallow baking dish, mix tomatoes, ¼ C. of the parsley, oregano and red pepper flakes.
2. Arrange the tilapia fillets over the tomato mixture in a single layer and drizzle with the lemon juice.
3. Place some tomato mixture over the tilapia fillets and sprinkle with the feta cheese evenly. Bake for about 12-14 minutes. Serve hot with the garnishing of remaining parsley.

Nutrition:

246 Calories

9.4g Carbohydrates

37.2g Protein

Quick Dinner Tilapia

Preparation Time: 15 minutes

Cooking Time: 6 minutes

Servings: 5

Ingredients:

- 2 tbsp. coconut oil
- 5 (5-oz.) tilapia fillets
- 2 tbsp. unsweetened coconut, shredded
- 3 garlic cloves, minced
- 1 tbsp. fresh ginger, minced
- 2 tbsp. low-sodium soy sauce
- 8 scallions, chopped

Directions:

1. Heat up coconut oil over medium heat and cook the tilapia fillets for about 2 minutes. Flip the side and stir in the coconut, garlic and ginger.
2. Cook for about 1 minute. Add the soy sauce and cook for about 1 minute. Add the scallions and cook for about 1-2 more minutes. Remove from heat and serve hot.

Nutrition:

189 Calories

4.4g Carbohydrates

27.7g Protein

Hit Salmon Dinner

Preparation Time: 15 minutes

Cooking Time: 20 minutes

Servings: 2

Ingredients:

- 1 C. walnuts
- 1 tbsp. fresh dill, chopped
- 2 tbsp. fresh lemon rind, grated
- ½ tsp. garlic salt
- 1 tbsp. butter, melted
- 3-4 tbsp. Dijon mustard
- 4 (3-oz.) salmon fillets
- 4 tsp. fresh lemon juice

Directions:

1. Preheat the oven to 3500 F. Line a large baking sheet with parchment paper. In a food processor, place the walnuts and pulse until chopped roughly. Add the dill, lemon rind, garlic salt, black pepper, and butter and pulse until a crumbly mixture form.
2. Place the salmon fillets onto prepared baking sheet in a single layer, skin-side down. Rub the top of each salmon fillet with Dijon mustard.

3. Place the walnut mixture over each fillet and gently, press into the surface of salmon. Bake for about 15-20 minutes. Remove the salmon fillets from oven and transfer onto the serving plates. Drizzle with the lemon juice and serve.

Nutrition:

691 Calories

10.3g Carbohydrates

49.8g Protein

Luscious Salmon

Preparation Time: 10 minutes

Cooking Time: 20 minutes

Servings: 2

Ingredients:

- ¼ C. cream cheese, softened
- 2 tbsp. fresh chives, chopped
- 1 tsp. garlic powder
- ¼ tsp. cayenne pepper
- 2 (4-oz.) salmon fillets

Directions:

1. Preheat the oven to 3500 F. Lightly, grease a small baking dish. In a bowl, add the cream cheese, chives, spices, salt and black pepper and mix well. Arrange the salmon fillets into prepared baking dish and top with the cream cheese mixture evenly.
2. Bake for about 15-20 minutes. Remove the salmon fillets from oven and serve hot.

Nutrition:

257 Calories

2.1g Carbohydrates

24.6g Protein

Insanely Simple Salmon

Preparation Time: 10 minutes

Cooking Time: 14 minutes

Servings: 4

Ingredients:

- 2 garlic cloves, minced
- 1 tbsp. fresh lemon zest, grated
- 2 tbsp. butter, melted
- 2 tbsp. fresh lemon juice
- 4 (6-oz.) skinless, boneless salmon fillets
- black pepper, to taste
- Salt
- 4 tbsp. feta cheese, crumbled

Directions:

1. Preheat the grill to medium-high heat. Grease the grill grate. Incorporate all ingredients except salmon fillets and feta and mix well. Add the salmon fillets and coat with garlic mixture generously.
2. Grill the salmon fillets for about 6-7 minutes per side. Serve immediately with the topping of feta.

Nutrition:

306 Calories

1.4g Carbohydrates

34.6g Protein

Entertaining Salmon

Preparation Time: 20 minutes

Cooking Time: 16 minutes

Servings: 4

Ingredients:

For Salmon:

- 4 (6-oz.) skinless salmon fillets
- 2 tbsp. fresh lemon juice
- 2 tbsp. olive oil, divided
- 1 tbsp. unsalted butter

For Filling:

- 4 oz. cream cheese, softened
- ¼ C. Parmesan cheese, grated finely
- 4 oz. frozen spinach thawed and squeezed
- 2 tsp. garlic, minced

Directions:

1. Season each salmon fillet then, drizzle with lemon juice and 1 tbsp. of oil. Arrange the salmon fillets onto a smooth surface.
2. With a sharp knife, cut a pocket into each salmon fillet about ¾ of the way through.
3. For filling: in a bowl, add the cream cheese, Parmesan cheese, spinach, garlic, salt and black pepper and mix well.

4. Place about 1-2 tbsp. of spinach mixture into each salmon pocket and spread evenly.
5. In a skillet, heat the remaining oil and butter over medium-high heat and cook the salmon fillets for about 6-8 minutes per side.
6. Remove the salmon fillets from heat and transfer onto the serving plates. Serve.

Nutrition:

438 Calories

2.4g Carbohydrates

38.1g Protein

Flavors Infused Salmon

Preparation Time: 15 minutes

Cooking Time: 15 minutes

Servings: 2

Ingredients:

- 2 (6-oz.) salmon fillets
- 2 streaky bacon slices
- 4 tbsp. pesto

Directions:

1. Preheat the oven to 3500 F. Line a medium baking sheet with parchment paper. Wrap each salmon fillet with 1 bacon slice and then, secure with a wooden skewer.
2. Place 2 tbsp. of pesto in the center of each salmon fillet. Arrange the salmon fillets onto prepared baking sheet. Bake for about 15 minutes.
3. Remove the salmon fillets from oven and serve hot.

Nutrition:

517 Calories

2.4g Carbohydrates

46.7g Protein:

Tuna Fish Salad

Preparation Time: 5 minutes

Cooking Time: 10 minutes

Servings: 1

Ingredient:

- 10 kalamata olives, pitted
- 1 small zucchini sliced lengthwise
- ½ diced avocado
- 2 cups of mixed greens
- 1 large diced tomato
- 1 sliced green onion
- 1 can chunk light tuna in water
- ¼ cup fresh parsley, chopped
- ½ cup fresh mint, chopped
- 1 tbsp. extra virgin olive oil
- 1 tbsp. balsamic vinegar
- ¼ tsp. fine sea salt
- ¾ tsp. black pepper, cracked

Directions:

1. Grill the zucchini slices on each side for a few minutes or as desired. Once cooked, cut it into bite-size pieces. Grab a large bowl and just put all the ingredients together in the container, mixing them together.

2. Serve while still fresh. This salad would taste best if eaten immediately so try not to have any leftovers.

Nutrition:

563 calories

30.9g total fat

37.5g carbohydrates

Mozzarella Tuna Melt

Preparation Time: 10 minutes

Cooking Time: 10 minutes

Serving: 2

Ingredients

- 1 tablespoon olive oil
- 1/2 cup diced yellow onion
- 8 ounces canned tuna
- 1/4 cup mayonnaise
- 2 large eggs
- 2 ounces shredded mozzarella cheese
- 1 green onion

Directions

1. Warm-up oil in a skillet over medium heat. Cook onion for 5 minutes. Strain the tuna then flake it into the skillet and stir in remaining ingredients.
2. Season well and cook for 2 minutes or until the cheese melts. Top with sliced green onion to serve.

Nutrition:

110 calories

10g fat

26g protein

Crabmeat Egg Scramble with White Sauce

Preparation Time: 10 minutes

Cooking Time: 15 minutes

Serving: 2

Ingredients

- 1 tbsp. olive oil
- 4 eggs
- 4 oz. crabmeat

Sauce:

- ¾ cup crème fraiche
- ½ cup chives, chopped
- ½ tsp. garlic powder

Directions

1. Scourge eggs with a fork in a bowl, and season with salt and black pepper.
2. Set a sauté pan over medium heat and warm olive oil. Add in the eggs and scramble them.
3. Stir in crabmeat and cook until cooked thoroughly. In a mixing dish, combine crème fraiche and garlic powder. Season with salt and sprinkle with chives. Serve the eggs with the white sauce.

Nutrition:

105 calories

9g fat

31g protein

Tuna Pickle Boats

Preparation Time: 40 minutes

Cooking Time: 0 minute

Serving: 4

Ingredients

- 1 (5-oz) can tuna, drained
- 2 large dill pickles
- ¼ tsp. lemon juice
- 2 tsp. mayonnaise
- ¼ tbsp. onion flakes
- 1 tsp. dill. chopped

Directions

1. Cut the pickles in half lengthwise. Spoon out the seeds to create boats; set aside.
2. Combine the mayonnaise, tuna, onion flakes, and lemon juice in a bowl. Fill each boat with tuna mixture. Sprinkle with dill and place in the fridge for 30 minutes before serving.

Nutrition:

311 calories

12g fat

4g protein

Salmon Salad with Lettuce & Avocado

Preparation Time: 5 minutes

Cooking Time: 0 minute

Serving: 3

Ingredients

- 2 slices smoked salmon
- 1 tsp. onion flakes
- 3 tbsp. mayonnaise
- 1 cup romaine lettuce
- 1 tbsp. lime juice
- 1 tbsp. extra virgin olive oil
- ½ avocado, sliced

Directions

1. Combine the salmon, mayonnaise, lime juice, olive oil, and salt in a small bowl; mix to combine well.
2. In a salad platter, arrange the shredded lettuce and onion flakes. Spread the salmon mixture over; top with avocado slices and serve.

Nutrition:

112 calories

6g fat

28g protein

Mackerel Lettuce Cups

Preparation Time: 10 minutes

Cooking Time: 20 minutes

Serving: 4

Ingredients

- 2 mackerel fillets
- 1 tbsp. olive oil
- 2 eggs
- 1 ½ cups water
- 1 tomato, seeded
- 2 tbsp. mayonnaise
- ½ head green lettuce

Directions

1. Preheat a grill pan over medium heat. Dash mackerel fillets with olive oil, and sprinkle with salt and black pepper. Add the fish to the preheated grill pan and cook on both sides for 6-8 minutes.
2. Bring the eggs to boil in salted water in a pot over medium heat for 10 minutes. Then, run the eggs in cold water, peel, and chop into small pieces. Transfer to a salad bowl.
3. Remove the mackerel fillets to the salad bowl. Include the tomatoes and mayonnaise; mix

evenly with a spoon. Layer two lettuce leaves each as cups and fill with two tablespoons of egg salad each.

Nutrition:

107 calories

14g fat

27g protein

Watercress & Shrimp Salad with Lemon Dressing

Preparation Time: 10 minutes

Cooking Time: 1 hour 10 minutes

Serving: 2

Ingredients

- 1 cup watercress leaves
- 2 tbsp. capers
- ½ pound shrimp
- 1 tbsp. dill

Dressing:

- ¼ cup mayonnaise
- ½ tsp. apple cider vinegar
- ¼ tsp. sesame seeds
- 1 tbsp. lemon juice
- 2 tsp. stevia

Directions

1. Combine the watercress leaves, shrimp, and dill in a large bowl. Whisk together the mayonnaise, vinegar, sesame seeds, black pepper, stevia, and lemon juice in another bowl. Season with salt.
2. Drizzle dressing over and gently toss to combine; refrigerate for 1 hour. Top with capers to serve.

Nutrition:

101 calories

8g fat

21g protein

Salad of Prawns and Mixed Lettuce Greens

Preparation Time: 10 minutes

Cooking Time: 15 minutes

Serving: 3

Ingredients

- 2 cups mixed lettuce greens
- ¼ cup aioli
- 1 tbsp. olive oil
- ½ pound tiger prawns
- ½ tsp. Dijon mustard
- 1 tbsp. lemon juice

Directions

1. Season the prawns with salt and chili pepper. Fry in warm olive oil over medium heat for 3 minutes on each side until prawns are pink. Set aside. Add the aioli, lemon juice and mustard in a small bowl. Mix until smooth and creamy.
2. Place the mixed lettuce greens in a bowl and pour half of the dressing on the salad. Toss with 2 spoons until mixed, and add the remaining dressing. Divide salad among plates and serve with prawns.

Nutrition:

107 calories

4g fat

26g protein

Ketogenic Baked Salmon with Lemon and Butter

Preparation Time: 10 minutes

Cooking Time: 30 minutes

Servings: 3

Ingredients:

1-pound salmon

1 lemon

3 oz. butter

1 tablespoon olive oil

Ground black pepper and sea salt to taste.

Directions:

Grease a large-sized baking dish with the olive oil and preheat your oven to 400°F.

Place the salmon on the baking dish, preferably skin-side down. Generously season with pepper and salt to taste.

Thinly slice the lemon and place the slices over the salmon. Cover the fish with ½ of the butter, preferably in very thin slices.

Bake until the salmon flakes easily with a fork and is opaque, for 25 to 30 minutes, on middle rack.

Now, over moderate heat in a small saucepan; heat the remaining butter until it begins to bubble. Immediately remove the pan from heat; set aside and let cool a bit. Gently add in some of the freshly squeezed lemon juice.

Serve the cooked fish with some of the prepared lemon butter and enjoy.

Nutrition:

Calories: 576

Total Fat: 46g

Saturated Fat: 22g

Total Carbohydrates: 1.3g

Dietary Fiber: 0.4g

Sugars: 0.4g

Protein: 31g

Ketogenicgenic Spicy Oyster

Preparation Time: 10 minutes

Cooking Time: 5 minutes

Servings: 2

Ingredients:

12 oysters shucked.

1 tablespoon olive oil

7-8 basil leaves, fresh

1 tablespoon garlic chili paste.

1/8 teaspoon salt

Directions:

Combine olive oil with garlic chili paste and salt in a medium size mixing bowl; mix well.

Add oysters into the prepared sauce; turning them several times until thoroughly coated.

Create a bed for the oysters to cook by spreading the basil leaves out on an oven-safe dish.

Transfer the oysters and sauce over the bed of basil leaves, spreading them in a single layer on the dish.

Turn on the broiler over high heat.

Place the dish on top rack (approximately a few inches away from the broiler) and broil for a few minutes.

Once done; immediately remove them from the oven. Serve hot and enjoy.

Nutrition:

Calories: 102 kcal

Total Fat: 8g

Saturated Fat: 2.5g

Total Carbohydrates: 2g

Dietary Fiber: 0g

Sugars: 0.3g

Protein: 4g

Garlic Lime Mahi-Mahi

Preparation Time: 15 minutes

Cooking Time: 10 minutes + 30 minutes marinate

Servings: 4

Ingredients:

4 Mahi-Mahi filets (approximately 1 to 1 ¼ pounds)

Zest and juice of 1 large lime, fresh

¼ cup avocado oil

3 cloves garlic, minced.

1/8 teaspoon each of ground black pepper and fine grain sea salt

Directions:

For Marinade: Thoroughly combine the entire ingredients (except the filets) together in a small-sized mixing bowl. Pour the mixture on top of filets in a large zip-lock bag or large shallow dish. Let marinate for 30 minutes, at room temperature.

Pour the marinade into a large sauté pan (preferably with a cover) and heat it over medium heat. Once hot; carefully add the filets into the hot pan; cover and cook the filets for a couple of minutes, until cooked through.

Immediately remove the sauté pan from heat; set aside and let rest for 5 minutes, covered. Serve warm and enjoy.

Nutrition:

Calories: 248 kcal

Total Fat: 14g

Saturated Fat: 1.7g

Total Carbohydrates: 0.7g

Dietary Fiber: 0.1g

Sugars: 0g

Protein: 24g

Fish and Leek Sauté

Preparation Time: 15 minutes

Cooking Time: 10 minutes

Servings: 2

Ingredients:

1 leek, chopped.

2 trout fillets, diced (approximately 8 oz.)

1 tablespoon tamari soy sauce

1 teaspoon ginger, grated.

1 tablespoon avocado oil

Salt to taste

Directions:

Over moderate heat in a large skillet; heat the avocado oil until hot. Once done; add and sauté the chopped leek for a few minutes, until turn soften.

Immediately add the diced trout with grated ginger, tamari sauce and salt to taste.

Continue to sauté the trout until it is not translucent anymore and cooked through.

Serve immediately and enjoy.

Nutrition:

Calories: 175 kcal

Total Fat: 7.6g

Saturated Fat: 1.5g

Total Carbohydrates: 5.2g

Dietary Fiber: 0.8g

Sugars: 1.7g

Protein: 21g

Smoked Salmon Salad

Preparation Time: 5 minutes

Cooking Time: 0 minutes

Servings: 1

Ingredients:

2 oz. smoked salmon

1 lemon slice

4 olives

1 teaspoon pink peppercorns crushed lightly.

A handful of arugula salad leaves, fresh

Directions:

Place the olives and salad leaves into a large plate or shallow bowl.

Arrange the smoked salmon over the salad.

Sprinkle the top of smoked salmon with lightly crushed pink peppercorns.

Garnish your salad with a lemon slice; serve immediately and enjoy.

Nutrition:

Calories: 149 kcal

Total Fat: 5.2g

Saturated Fat: 1.4g

Total Carbohydrates: 4g

Dietary Fiber: 1.7g

Sugars: 3.4g

Protein: 11g

Ketogenic Baked Salmon with Pesto

Preparation Time: 10 minutes

Cooking Time: 30 minutes

Servings: 2

Ingredients:

1 oz. green pesto

½ pound salmon

Pepper and salt to taste.

For Green sauce:

¼ cup Greek yogurt

1 oz. green pesto

¼ teaspoon garlic

Pepper and salt to taste.

Directions:

Preheat your oven to 400°F.

Arrange the salmon in a well-greased baking dish, preferably skin-side down. Spread the pesto over the salmon and then, sprinkle with pepper and salt to taste.

Bake in the preheated oven until the salmon flakes easily with a fork, for 25 to 30 minutes.

In the meantime, stir the entire sauce ingredients together in a large bowl. Serve the cooked fish with some of the prepared sauce and enjoy.

Nutrition:

Calories: 274 kcal

Total Fat: 21g

Saturated Fat: 3.9g

Total Carbohydrates: 2.9g

Dietary Fiber: 0.6g

Sugars: 1.7g

Protein: 26g

Roasted Salmon with Parmesan Dill Crust

Preparation Time: 10 minutes

Cooking Time: 10 minutes

Servings: 2

Ingredients:

½ pound salmon; cut into pieces.

1 tablespoon dill weed.

¼ cup cottage cheese

1 tablespoon olive oil

¼ cup parmesan cheese, grated.

Directions:

Preheat your oven to 450°F.

Combine cottage cheese with parmesan cheese, olive oil and dill in a large-sized mixing bowl; mix well.

Line a large-sized baking sheet with aluminum foil and then, arrange the salmon pieces on it.

Smear ½ of the cottage cheese mix over the salmon.

Roast in the preheated oven until the fish flakes easily and crust is brown, for 10 minutes.

Serve the cooked fish with the remaining prepared sauce and enjoy.

Nutrition:

Calories: 352 kcal

Total Fat: 22g

Saturated Fat: 6.6g

Total Carbohydrates: 5.7g

Dietary Fiber: 1.5g

Sugars: 0.5g

Protein: 33g

Ketogenic Fried Salmon with Broccoli and Cheese

Preparation Time: 15 minutes

Cooking Time: 25 minutes

Servings: 3

Ingredients:

¾ pound salmon; cut into pieces.

3 tablespoons butter

½ pound broccoli; cut into small florets.

2 oz. cheddar cheese, grated.

Pepper and salt to taste.

1 lime

Directions:

Preheat your oven using the broiler settings, to 400°F.

Let the broccoli florets to simmer for a couple of minutes, preferably in lightly salted water. Ensure that the broccoli maintains its delicate color and chewy texture; drain well.

Now arrange the broccoli in a baking dish, preferably well-greased. Add butter and pepper to taste.

Sprinkle with cheese and bake in the preheated oven until the cheese turns golden in color, for 15 to 20 minutes.

Now, over moderate heat in a large saucepan; heat the butter until completely melted and fry the salmon pieces for a couple of minutes per side. Serve the pan-fried salmon with baked broccoli and enjoy.

Nutrition:

Calories: 392g

Total Fat: 25g

Saturated Fat: 11.8g

Total Carbohydrates: 5.8g

Dietary Fiber: 3.4g

Sugars: 1.4g

Protein: 31g

Breakfast Potatoes

Preparation Time: 15 minutes

Cooking Time: 15 minutes

Serving: 2

Ingredients:

- 4 gold potatoes, washed and peeled
- Water as needed
- 1 tbsp. bacon fat or butter
- 2 tsp. Italian seasoning
- Salt and pepper to taste
- 1 cup chives, chopped for serving

Directions:

1. Place the potatoes in the Instant Pot and pour the water to cover them. Close and lock the lid. Select MANUAL and cook at HIGH pressure for 10 minutes. Once cooking is complete, select CANCEL and let Naturally Release for 10 minutes. Release any remaining steam manually. Uncover the pot.
2. Transfer the potatoes to a bowl and mash them a bit with a fork. Select the SAUTÉ setting on the Instant Pot, add the bacon fat and heat up. Return the mashed potatoes to the pot, add the Italian seasoning, salt and pepper, stir well.

3. Close and lock the lid. Select MANUAL and cook at HIGH pressure for 1 minute. When the timer goes off, use a Quick Release. Carefully open the lid. Stir the potatoes and top with chives. Serve.

Nutrition:

128 Calories

0.2g Fat

3.1g Protein

29.9g Carbohydrates

Potato Breakfast Hash

Preparation Time: 15 minutes

Cooking Time: 5 minutes

Serving: 4

Ingredients:

- 2 medium onion, chopped
- 2 cloves garlic, minced
- 2 large sweet potato, diced into 1-inch pieces
- 2 large potato, diced into ½ inch pieces
- 4 bell peppers, chopped
- 2 tbsp. olive oil
- 1 tsp. kosher salt
- ½ tsp. black pepper
- 1½ tsp. of paprika
- 1½ tsp. cumin
- ¼ tsp. cayenne pepper
- 1 cup water

Directions:

1. In the Instant Pot, combine the onion, garlic, sweet potato, potato, bell peppers, and oil. Season with salt, pepper, paprika, cumin, and cayenne pepper. Mix well. Pour in the water. Close and lock the lid.

2. Select MANUAL and cook at HIGH pressure for 1 minutes. When the timer beeps, use a Quick Release. Carefully unlock the lid. Select SAUTÉ and cook the mixture for about 7 minutes, until the potatoes start to brown.
3. Press the CANCEL key to stop the SAUTÉ function. Serve warm.

Nutrition:

238 Calories

34.9g Carbohydrates

9.6g Protein

7.4g Fat

Tasty Potato Hash

Preparation Time: 15 minutes

Cooking Time: 10 minutes

Serving: 4-6

Ingredients:

- 1 tbsp. olive oil
- 5 medium potatoes, peeled and roughly chopped
- 5 eggs, whisked
- 1 cup cheddar cheese, shredded
- 1 cup ham, chopped
- ¼ cup water
- Salt and ground black pepper to the taste

Directions:

1. Select the SAUTÉ setting on the Instant Pot and heat the oil. Add the potatoes and sauté for 3-4 minutes, until slightly brown.
2. Add eggs, cheese, ham, water, salt and pepper. Stir well. Close and lock the lid. Press the CANCEL button to stop the SAUTE function, then select the MANUAL setting and set the cooking time for 5 minutes at HIGH pressure.

3. Once pressure cooking is complete, select CANCEL and use a Quick Release. Carefully unlock the lid. Serve warm.

Nutrition:

198 Calories

0.7g Fat

4g Protein

Baked Potatoes

Preparation Time: 10 minutes

Cooking Time: 30 minutes

Serving: 8

Ingredients:

- 5 lbs. potatoes, peeled and cut into half
- 1½ cups water
- Salt to taste

Directions:

1. Prepare the Instant Pot by adding the water to the pot and placing the steamer basket in it. Place the potatoes in the basket. Close and secure the lid.
2. Select the MANUAL setting and set the cooking time for 10 minutes at HIGH pressure. Once cooking is complete, let the pressure Release Naturally for 15 minutes. Release any remaining steam manually. Uncover the pot. Season with salt and serve.

Nutrition:

110 Calories

26g Carbohydrate

2g Fiber

0g Fat

Whole Baked Potatoes

Preparation Time: 10 minutes

Cooking Time: 25 minutes

Servings: 4-6

Ingredients:

- 6-8 medium Russet potatoes
- ½ tsp. kosher salt
- ½ tsp. ground black pepper
- 2 tbsp. olive oil
- 1 cup water

Directions:

1. Wash the potatoes and pat dry. Using a fork, pierce the middle of each potato. In a bowl, combine the salt, pepper and oil. Mix well.
2. Add the potatoes to the bowl and brush them well with the mixture. Pour the water into the Instant Pot and set a steam rack in the pot. Place the potatoes on the steam rack. Close and lock the lid.
3. Select MANUAL and cook at HIGH pressure for 10 minutes. Once timer goes off, use a Quick Release. Carefully unlock the lid. Transfer the potatoes to a serving bowl. Serve with butter and fresh dill.

Nutrition:

110 Calories

26g Carbohydrates

2g Fiber

0g Fat

Crispy Potatoes

Preparation Time: 20 minutes

Cooking Time: 30 minutes

Serving: 4

Ingredients:

- 2 tbsp. olive oil
- 2 tbsp. butter
- 1½ lbs. Yukon gold potatoes, cut in half
- 1 tsp. sea salt
- 1 tsp. ground black pepper
- ½ cup water or broth

Directions:

1. Select the SAUTÉ setting on the Instant Pot and heat the oil. Add the butter and melt it. Add the potatoes and sauté, stirring occasionally, for 10 minutes until the halves have turned slightly golden.
2. Season with salt and pepper, stir well. Pour in the water. Close and lock the lid.
3. Press the CANCEL button to reset the cooking program, then press the MANUAL button and set the cooking time for 6 minutes at HIGH pressure. Once cooking is complete, select CANCEL and let Naturally Release for 20

minutes. Release any remaining steam manually. Uncover the pot.
4. Taste for seasoning and add more salt if needed. Serve.

Nutrition:

182 Calories

29g Carbohydrates

4.5g Fiber

3.4g Protein

Herb Roasted New Potatoes

Preparation Time: 15 minutes

Cooking Time: 15 minutes

Serving: 4

Ingredients:

- 3 tbsp. olive oil
- 1½ - 2 lbs. small Yukon gold or red potatoes
- ½ tsp. garlic powder
- ½ tsp. dried marjoram
- ½ tsp. dried thyme
- ½ tsp. dried oregano
- ¼ tsp. dried rosemary
- 1 tsp. sea salt
- ½ tsp. ground black pepper
- ½ cup chicken broth or water

Directions:

1. Rinse the potatoes and pat dry with a kitchen paper. Preheat the Instant Pot by selecting SAUTÉ. Add and heat the oil.
2. Add the potatoes and cook, stirring occasionally, for 6-7 minutes until the potatoes have turned light brown and crisp. Poke some holes using a fork. You may have to cook the potatoes in two batches.

3. In a bowl, combine the garlic powder, marjoram, thyme, oregano, rosemary, salt, and pepper. Add the herb mix to the pot and stir well. Pour in the water. Close and lock the lid.
4. Press the CANCEL button to stop the SAUTE function, then select the MANUAL setting and set the cooking time for 7 minutes at HIGH pressure. Once timer goes off, use a Quick Release. Carefully unlock the lid.
5. Taste for seasoning and add more salt if needed. Serve.

Nutrition:

390 Calories

32g Total Fats

3g protein

3.1g Fiber

Mashed Potatoes

Preparation Time: 10 minutes

Cooking Time: 35 minutes

Serving: 4-6

Ingredients:

- 2 lbs. potatoes, peeled and quartered
- 1 cup water
- 1 cup milk
- 3 tbsp. butter
- Salt and ground black pepper to taste

Directions:

1. Pour the water into the Instant Pot and insert a steamer basket. Put the potatoes in the basket.
2. Close and lock the lid. Select the MANUAL setting and set the cooking time for 15 minutes at HIGH pressure. Once cooking is complete, use a Natural Release for 15 minutes, and then release any remaining pressure manually. Open the lid.
3. Transfer the potatoes to a bowl. Add the milk and butter. Mash until creamy and smooth. Season with salt and pepper. Serve.

Nutrition:

232 Calories

1.6g Fat

9.6g Protein

48g Carbohydrates

www.ingramcontent.com/pod-product-compliance
Lightning Source LLC
Chambersburg PA
CBHW070723030426
42336CB00013B/1908